Confessions
of a Caregiver

Joseph Skillin ● ● ● ● ● ● ● ● ● ●

Confessions
of a Caregiver

When Alzheimer's
Comes to Your Home

● ●

TATE PUBLISHING & *Enterprises*

Published by Tate Publishing & Enterprises, LLC
127 E. Trade Center Terrace | Mustang, Oklahoma 73064 USA
1.888.361.9473 | www.tatepublishing.com

Tate Publishing is committed to excellence in the publishing industry. The company reflects the philosophy established by the founders, based on Psalm 68:11,
"The Lord gave the word and great was the company of those who published it."

Book design copyright © 2009 by Tate Publishing, LLC. All rights reserved.
Cover design by Tyler Evans
Interior design by Stephanie Woloszyn

Published in the United States of America

ISBN: 978-1-60799-503-6
1. Health & Fitness / Diseases / Alzheimer's & Dementia
2. Self-Help / Stress Management
09.03.11

This book is dedicated to

● ●

Donna, an angel sent to us.

And Tim, another angel, far away, but in touch daily.

TABLE OF CONTENTS

Foreword

● ●

This book has a single purpose. I expose my own feelings so that you can prepare yourself to undergo the same harsh, demanding array of feelings when you find yourself living with and caring for an Alzheimer's patient.

This book is not about a disease. It is mainly about the feelings of a man living with someone who has Alzheimer's.

This book is about the complex feelings you will experience when Alzheimer's comes to your home—when you decide to take care of your mother, your father, or your spouse who has been stricken with this insidious disease.

There are about six million people diagnosed with Alzheimer's disease in this country. Many are taken care of at home; perhaps in their own home; perhaps in the home of a daughter or son. Ten million Americans struggle to take care of a relative with Alzheimer's or some other form of dementia according to a series of articles in several June, 2007, issues of USA Today.

This book will not explain the clinical aspects of Alzheimer's; it will not describe how Alzheimer's will affect your loved one; it will not elaborate on the hundreds of resources to help you in caring for your loved one suffering from this hideous disease; it will not chronicle the daily events of my mother-in-law, who has Alzheimer's and is living in our house. It is, rather, about my feelings as I go through this experience.

My purpose is to share my own feelings about Alzheimer's so you may prepare yourself for similar feelings if your parent or spouse becomes a victim—if Alzheimer's comes to your home. Be prepared. Even be forewarned. Often it will be overwhelming.

Introduction

● ●

It really had started earlier—the confusion, the slowing down, the forgetting, the hesitation of speech and movement, but by the end of the summer we realized that my mother-in-law had Alzheimer's disease. My wife and I made the decision to take her in and give her care. I'm not sure we were prepared for the effects of this decision. No one explained what we were getting into.

My mother-in-law (whom I call Mom) has Alzheimer's and is living in our home. In fact, she has taken over our house! It seems that everything is focused on her or scheduled around her. Decisions are based on her—her needs and her illness.

My wife, Penny, and I were invited to dinner one Thursday night. The question was not whether we wanted to go. It was whether we *could* go. *Could we get someone to watch Mom? Could we stay long, or would we need to get back home to let the caregiver go home?*

A small, insignificant decision? Sure. But when virtually every decision follows that same pattern, it becomes frustrating and maddening. It leads to feelings of resentment.

And it's the same with big and truly significant decisions. Mom has been living with us for eight years. During this period, for several reasons, it has seemed a good time to move. I remember the first discussion, six years ago. "This would be a perfect time to move. The house is starting to need some repairs ... mortgage rates are low ... people want to move into this neighborhood ... we know about six places we could move to and be really happy."

"Yeah, but what about Mom? How would she do in a strange place? I'm not sure it would be good for her ... Maybe we should just wait and see what happens with her." And thus we have waited, watching the mortgage rates go up, and passing on what seemed a few excellent opportunities to move.

My reactive feelings to this Alzheimer's-in-the-house situation are all over the place: confusing, positive and negative, unclear and contradictory, hopeful and pessimistic, loving and resentful.

Sometimes I feel like screaming in frustration. Other times I say, "This is just the way it is. You take care of family. You love. And you do it with a generous heart and a certain amount of joy."

In this book, you'll see the ups and downs and all sides of the absolute craziness the disease called Alzheimer's brings into your house. You'll get a little glimpse of what it does to Mom so you'll know what to expect. But mostly you'll see how it affects the caregiver so you'll be prepared for your own feelings. You'll see how it brings out the very best in my wife and my children, so you'll see why I say there is good in all this.

You'll see the negative, the sad, and the frustrating. But you'll also see the positive, the love, the hope, and the rewards. It's as if someone picked up the magnificent kaleidoscope off my desk and painted several of the brilliant pieces of glass a matt black. The darkness is there—no doubt, but so are the many beautiful reds, yellows, greens, blues, and oranges. I still can control the rotation of the glasses to focus on what I want to see. Even though it is difficult at times, I can find the colorful pieces and enjoy their beauty.

Alzheimer's, if it comes to your home, will present you with a kaleidoscope of experiences and feelings. Be ready to find heroes in the daily difficulties. You will laugh; you will cry. You will see true love and feel frustration. You will lose patience; you will be forced to calm down. You will dislike what the disease does, yet it will prepare you for your own future.

Walk with me through these pages as I portray what I've felt during this process. My purpose is to prepare you for your own experiences with Alzheimer's in the house. When you get to glimpse where I've been, perhaps you won't feel quite so frustrated or guilty. You will fully realize that many others have been there before you, or are there even today. You'll feel normal rather than unusual, connected rather than isolated, familiar rather than uncertain, maybe even confident rather than scared.

At the end of each section, I've written a prayer—a

simple, honest, eyes-closed, sincere prayer spoken to God. These prayers are not just written productions to add something to this book. They are honest words expressing my heart to God. If you relate to them, make them your own.

Or just speak your own heart to God. It helps, and he helps.

A Prayer for Assurance

God of Abraham, Isaac, and Jacob, be with me now. I need your help. I need your assurances.

Just as you spent forty years walking with your people in the desert, walk with me as I wrestle with this illness called Alzheimer's. I'm not the one with the disease, but I'm going to care for the one who has it. I know that at times it will try my patience and even change my life. At times it will be my desert—barren, dry, relentless.

So be with me. Even more, *assure* me that you are with me. Give me signs of your presence. Let me feel the warmth of your love, the gentleness of your touch, and the strength of your power. I want to see you, Lord. As I take this uncharted journey of caring for an Alzheimer's patient, assure me of your presence and encourage me with your power.

Amen.

How I Feel

●●●●●●●●●●●●●●●●●●●●●●●●●●●●●

I feel resentful. I feel sad. I feel loving. I feel dutiful. I feel helpful. I feel satisfied. I feel all of the above at different times to different degrees. Feelings which at times are separate and at times conjoined.

My Negative Feelings

The negative feelings I most easily identify in myself are resentment, anger, sadness, and frustration.

• I Feel Resentful

Sometimes I feel resentment. I suspect that resentment is a feeling more pervasive in the in-law of an Alzheimer's patient than it is in the son or daughter. If your mom or dad gets Alzheimer's, that's hard enough and very difficult to handle every day. But filial love kicks in and helps you rise to the occasion and sustain that level of care for months and years. It's your mom or dad, and you feel the need and even some desire to care for them.

But if it is your mother-in-law, as in my case, negative feelings come more easily. Often, I feel resentment. I feel like I've lost what is dear to me—a simple life with my wife, the way we planned and imagined it, the two of us with a lot of freedom now that the children are grown and gone. But it is not just the two of us in a mature autumnal life of quiet love and leisurely activity; rather it is a life busier and more hampered than it has ever been.

It is busier. Primarily, it is busier for my wife. But because we're married in heart and spirit as well as on paper, we share things—thoughts, goals, values, and chores. So while Penny has additional tasks in her daily life while caring for her mom, I have additional chores just in doing more of the ordinary and routine tasks around the house. To ease my wife's busy schedule, I'll now do more of the laundry, dishwashing, emptying the dishwasher, setting the table, vacuuming, etc. I don't state this looking for sympathy. It's just a fact. Alzheimer's changes everything in the home.

Normally chaos reigns supreme. There are times when Mom has the TV blaring, when one caregiver is coming in and another is going out, when someone else is coming in to help with some cleaning. While I appreciate the real help these people provide, my soul, naturally seeking tranquility, says, "All of you get out of here. I want my house back."

Our life is busier. And it is more hampered. When we do go out socially, we often leave early, telling our host that we have to get back for our "babysitter." Of course, it's not really a babysitter but a caregiver. We're grateful that the caregiver stays late on occasion so we can get away. But, on the other hand, we need to respect her needs and let her get home to her own family and spend time with them.

Comparing Mom's caregiver to a babysitter has some genuine parallels, but there is one enormous difference. It is relatively easy to find a babysitter, and one's baby usually doesn't care too much who it is. But you can't get just anyone to watch an Alzheimer's patient when you want to duck out for an evening! There are not too many people willing to care for such a patient for even a few hours in one evening. More importantly, it is the patient who will balk. He or she so often reacts negatively to a stranger and won't feel comfortable, which causes acting out. Your evening will be ruined before you've even had a chance to get out of the house.

No question about it. Our life is more hampered, because our social and leisure schedule is secondary to her care and the schedule of her caregivers. To wit, Penny and I have been to a movie no more than four times in the last two years. That might seem unrealistic, but it is just plain difficult to arrange to get away for leisurely enjoyment.

There are times when I don't know if I'm angry, resentful, or guilty—or all three at once! One Thursday, a beautiful early summer day, the sun, not yet too hot, was calling the world to come outside and enjoy life. I got the urge to take Penny up the street for a latté. We would sit outside, talk a little, look a lot, hold hands, and just enjoy the simple experience. I went upstairs to suggest the idea (I work out of my house) and Penny was in a serious conversation with the caregiver. I just knew this was not the appropriate time to suggest sitting around sipping *lattes*. So I just said a feeble, "Hi." And went back down to my office.

Occasionally, I want to take Penny to lunch on the

spur of the moment, or just go out to dinner, or plan a spontaneous weekend away. But I get held up by the fact that she can't just leave her mom at a moment's notice and go with me. So I don't go. I feel some resentment. To myself I say, "I want my freedom back. I want my life back. I want my wife back."

An Alzheimer's parent in the house does force change to the reality and the vision of your marriage. Just the other day, Penny verbalized her concern that this whole situation is "at the expense of our marriage." Our focus on each other is lessened because of our need to focus on Mom. Our private time together is lessened because of the time focused on her and the time interrupted by caregivers coming and going all times of night and day. Our focus on each other is lessened by the frequent exhaustion that overcomes my wife so many nights after being with her mother all day.

I hastened to assure Penny that Mom's presence is not at the expense of our marriage. I countered that, as long as we can get one good laugh every night before we go to bed, our marriage will be good, will survive, and will even get stronger. At times, we both feel that this whole situation is killing our marriage. But, fortunately, we know better. Our marriage is not deteriorating. If anything it is getting stronger. There are some strains on it, but our love is more powerful than they are.

But let's be real about those strains. There are many times when I want my wife's attention and it's not available. She needs to deal with her mother, or the caregiver, or a nurse, or take her to a doctor's appointment. My mature self understands this, accepts this, and even admires it. But my weaker side, nonetheless, says, "I want my wife back."

I know that resentment comes only to the degree that I am being selfish and childish. I'm smart enough to know that long-range realities do not usually turn out the way one plans them. I should spend more time trying to help my wife and her mother and less time concerned about what I'm missing.

A Prayer in Anger

God, I have to be honest. You already know my heart and have read my soul, so I may as well speak frankly.

Today I am in a poor-me-pity-me mood. I hate the fact that this sickness is in my life and that I'm stuck with caring for it. I resent that the illness even exists. I resent that it consumes my mother-in-law. I resent that it intrudes on our family. I resent that it intrudes on my life.

I don't want it. I don't want to deal with it. I don't want it to continue.

I'm mad at everybody and everything. I'm just in a terrible, rotten mood.

Amen.

• I Feel Sad

It's sad to watch Mom. She's slowly dying. Yes, we all are; but with her I can see it, hear it, watch it, and feel it. Some days she looks like 20 percent of her soul left her last night. Even though I know she is physically strong, at times I think she could die today or tonight. It is sad to watch an able body lose its mind, slowly, daily, as if it is no more than evaporating water.

As I watch her struggle with basic mental experiences—recognition, understanding, memory, and expression—I feel a sadness that I have never attributed to my own life. Yes, I have witnessed many a sad event in my life, but never has a slow, daily, human deterioration been this visible or been such a constant environment of my life. It is hard for me to watch. How much more terrible must it be for her in those moments when she lapses into full recognition of her state!

One evening I was in the kitchen, Mom was in the family room on the sofa supposedly watching television. I looked over at her and was struck by what a strange and sad picture I was witnessing. Outwardly she looked normal—attractively dressed, tastefully done cosmetics, hair nicely brushed. But I realized I was observing a person standing at the edge of the river Styx. She watched TV without seeing it; she listened without hearing the noise. She was not asleep, but not awake either. She had no energy, but was not tired. She was in some strange state that seemed to be self-absorption without self-recognition. She lives in the mysterious, haunting, and cruel world of Alzheimer's.

There are two forms of sadness relative to Alzheimer's. There is sadness for someone you love, and there is sadness for oneself when you realize that this person you love is disappearing from your life.

I am reminded of my own mother when she began her dismal journey through the agonies of Alzheimer's. She started with exasperation. "Fiddlesticks!" she would curse. (This obviously was a long time ago, when real swearing was not the norm.) "Why can't I remember that name?!" Exasperation gave way to embarrassment, embarrassment to silence, silence to withdrawal, and withdrawal to rapid and obvious physical deterioration. The entire process of wearing away continued for years as a slow but defiant process of gradual death. I watched in sadness as my mother morphed from a vibrant, proud, and loving mother to a hesitant, reluctant, and unconfident loner—to a little old lady who didn't know my name, to a catatonic shell of a body with no mind and only half her soul. How sad it felt to witness this. Part of the sadness was in seeing her personal struggles as she went through this. Part was my own personal sadness in realizing that my mother was dying. A double-edged sword.

Penny says of her mom: "It's sad. She's dying, slowly but really. It's sad to watch her dying every day." Penny's sadness is not for herself. Neither is mine. It is for her mother. There are many moments, even full days, when Mom knows she is sick, confused, and limited in her capacities. This was a vibrant, often laughing, busy woman who enjoyed so many things in her life. And she sees this all ripped away from her, denied her, today. This is what is sad: to watch her falling into physical, emotional, and mental quicksand, knowing she is being swallowed up and will not escape.

A Prayer of Sadness

I think of Mom when I first met her—pretty, smiling, confident, energetic, and full of fun. I see her now—absent all these qualities.

Lord, I look at all creation and see a pattern: everything deteriorates, wears out, breaks down, gets used up, and ultimately stops, disappears, or dies.

As a Christian, I believe in the final triumph of good over evil, life over death, and the ultimate perfection of life. But meanwhile, in this life that some call a vale of tears, there is so much sadness conceived of loss. I remember when my first dog, Wolf, got killed. I just sat on the curb, held her in my arms, and refused to leave her and go home. I just cried and cried. There have been other pets in my life and other losses that have brought tears and sadness. This one—watching Mom whither away—is different, Lord. It is a sadness that stretches from day to day while watching a body deteriorate and a soul disappear. This is so sad.

Hug me, God. I feel empty inside.

Amen.

• I Feel Frustrated

Mom wears two hearing aids. She keeps taking them out. When I try to talk to her, she can't hear me.

This is frustrating.

The TV volume is as loud as Daytona. I give her back her hearing aids and turn down the volume of the TV. She removes the hearing aids, and, of course, the volume goes back up. This is frustrating.

I went to Radio Shack and purchased a hearing assistance set for her. It's like a Wi-Fi between the TV sound system and a set of well padded, comfortable headphones she could wear. It allows her to turn up the volume as high as she wants, without flooding the room with the noise. I thought this private sound system would be perfect for her and relief for me. She put them on for ten minutes the first day and then refused to use them any more. Refused. So, of course, the volume again is constantly at Daytona decibels.

This is frustrating.

Penny goes out of her way to make Mom look attractive. This means many moments brushing her hair, spraying it, making it just right. As soon as Mom sits in front of the TV, her first action is to run her hands through her hair in some random fashion that defies diagrams. But the result is always the same—her hair looks absolutely trashed!

This is frustrating.

Mom has a little toy poodle that sits on her lap much of the day. The dog barks loud and long at the slightest motion. I call to Mom to quiet her dog and she just looks at me with a distant, vacant stare. The dog continues barking.

This is frustrating.

Knowing that some exercise of the brain is good for anyone, I ask Mom, "Where did you go today?"

"Nowhere."

(Actually Penny took her to the store and they just walked back in with bags of groceries.)

"Didn't you go to the store?"

She responds, "No."

Penny chimes in, "Mom, we just came back from the store!"

Mom asks, "We did?"

This is frustrating.

In a moment of guilt or in an honest effort to get her engaged in anything for a moment, I'll try to make basic, light conversation with Mom. Or, knowing exercise is very important for her, I'll say, "Come on; let's take a little walk around the house."

"No. I don't want to."

And we both know that I can't make her do this.

This is frustrating.

It is frustrating when I can't seem to do anything about the noise.

More importantly, it is frustrating to want to help but be unable to do so.

Frustrating to want to extend the exercise of her talents, but being unable to.

It is frustrating to want to re-spark some dying ember in her soul, but being unable to.

It is frustrating to want to hold back the unstoppable, overwhelming lava-flow of this disease, while knowing she will never win. I will never win.

A Prayer When Frustrated

Wow, God! If I get this frustrated over these little things, by comparison,
You must get extremely frustrated!
You give me plenty of gifts that I squander.
You make my soul and spirit beautiful, and I mess them up.
You give me virtues to strengthen my soul, and I ignore them.
You even talk to me and I refuse to listen.

This has to be so frustrating to you.
But that is reducing you to human terms.
Fortunately, you are bigger than that, Lord.
You don't get frustrated. You just forgive and give more.
You are merciful, forgiving, lavish, and totally generous.
You don't focus on my negatives, but take me as I am.
You encourage me, but never reject me.
You see my weaknesses, but only offer me more gifts.

Give me some insight here, Lord.

Help me to stay a little more positive, a little less frustrated.

Help me to be a little more accepting of Alzheimer's environment, a little less frustrated by what does not coincide with my plan, a little more understanding of my patient's condition, a little more patient. Just a little. Just for today.

Amen.

• Identify Your Own Negative Feelings

What is the most common negative feeling you recognize in yourself as a caregiver?

_____

_____

_____

_____

Is it something you recognize at the time or only when you look back at the end of the day?

_____

_____

_____

_____

List all the negative feelings you see in yourself as a caregiver.

_____

_____

_____

_____

Now go back to that list you just made and try to identify the specific circumstances that trigger those negative feelings.

_____

_____

_____

_____

Can you think of ways to see those triggers coming and be prepared to choose a different feeling or different response in the future?

_____

_____

_____

_____

My Positive Feelings

•••••••••••••••••••••••••

The positive feelings and values that keep me going are love, duty, and helpfulness

• I Feel Loving

As much as I hate the disease, as much as I let myself be bothered by the TV blaring all day, as much as I resent the intrusions on my life because of this Alzheimer's-in-the-house, I love Mom and would do anything to help her.

Fortunately, I can rely on my wife to be the primary caregiver to her mom. I am truly grateful for that because I don't want to have to cook her breakfast, bathe her, dress her, take her to the bathroom, and listen to her when she makes absolutely no sense. Penny and some assisting caregivers attend to all that. Honestly, I'm thankful that I don't have the prime responsibility to do all those things.

I've never been comfortable around sick and feeble people. I elaborate on this in the chapter "What I Fear." For now, suffice it to say that I just don't want to be the one administering physical care. (I see this as a personal weakness, something to confront, to deal with, and to overcome. And I know I will.)

Even though I don't *do* those daily, necessary activities for Mom, I do love her. I know that if Penny had no help in caring for her, I would do more in the way of physically caring for her. If none of her family took care of her, I would. I know I love her and want what is best for her.

I don't communicate with Mom very well in the normal way—talking. She doesn't hear too well and she seems to pay very little attention to me when I talk to her. Perhaps it is because I don't try hard enough; perhaps it's because she has some jealousy toward me for stealing her daughter away long ago! I don't know why, and, really, I don't care. It's just a fact—we don't talk very much. I can't get a normal conversation going with her.

So I try to express my love to her in an unusual way. Sometimes it works; often it does not. But when it does, both Mom and I beam!

I try to get her to laugh. I believe laughter is good for the soul and a sign of vitality. I think laughter always contains a glimmer of hope and produces a moment of joy. So I try to make her laugh. That's my best expression of love for her. While some in the family think my humor is non-existent or crazy, Penny (usually) likes it. And if it's good enough for her, it can be good enough for her mother. It's all I have.

As evil as the sickness is or as difficult as the environment is, I love the woman at the center of it. I want comfort for her and any degree of happiness that can be created. I love her and want to share in bringing her that comfort and happiness. I have not succeeded in finding many ways to deliver on this desire, but this one works for me.

The love is there. The expression of that love is unusual. But it is honest. It is me; loving in my own crazy way.

A Prayer of Love

Lord, when you created us in your own image and likeness, when you breathed into us the very breath of your own life, you made us lovers. Thank you for this wonderful gift. Without love, I am nothing, with just an empty life of insignificance, sour relationships, useless goals, and false joy. With love, I can aspire to the heights of heaven, endure all things, create wonders in this world, share my abundance, and live in genuine joy.

This day, fill me with your spirit that I might help others.

This day, fill me with your love that I might care for Mom with joy.

This day, fill me with your patience that I might be more patient with her.

This day, fill me with your abundance that I might be generous with her.

Just this day, fill me with your forgiveness that I might not be exasperated with her.

Just this day, overwhelm my selfishness with the

power of your love, which is generous, patient, constant, forgiving, and all-consuming.

Just this day, help me to show my love to Mom and make her day a little more pleasant.

I need your love. God, speed your love to me.

Amen.

• I Feel Dutiful

When my own mother had Alzheimer's, she lived in California while I resided in Atlanta. We were born and raised in San Francisco, but in time all the family moved out of The City. My mother ended up in a nursing home in Stockton near my brother's place, where she lived the last five or six years of her fading life.

Whenever I flew to San Francisco, whether for business or pleasure, I drove down to see my mother in Stockton. I knew I would drive two hours to get there; go in to see her and have absolutely no conversation, perhaps not even a sparkle of recognition. I knew I would stay an awkward twenty or thirty minutes with no apparent communication. I would talk to her, feeling that she comprehended nothing of what I was saying. I'd kiss her, stroke her hair a bit, keep talking to her, and once even sang to her. I was never convinced that all this meant nothing. On the other hand, I was never convinced that she recognized any satisfaction from it. Every time I took this little extra trip, I was doubtful and confused. *Was this trip worth it? What good did it accomplish?*

I'd get back into my Avis or Hertz, usually hot now from baking in the Stockton sun, and ask myself, *Why did you come here? Two hours to get here, an empty visit, and now you have to drive two hours back again. Why do this?*

My answer was already in my heart. I did it because she was my mother. I did it because of that ever present combination of love and duty. I did it because that's what you do—you take care of those you love, do whatever you can, visit the ones you love, make a few sacrifices to show them the love they deserve.

Someone e-mailed me this story. It cited no source, but was entitled "In a Hurry." It has taught me how to give a more generous response to Alzheimer's.

It was a busy morning, about eight thirty, when an elderly gentleman in his eighties, arrived to have stitches removed from his thumb. He said he was in a hurry as he had an appointment at 9:00 am.

I took his vital signs and had him take a seat, knowing it would be over an hour before someone would to able to see him. I saw him looking at his watch and decided, since I was not busy with another patient, I would evaluate his wound.

On exam, it was well healed, so I talked to one of the doctors, got the needed supplies to remove his sutures, and began to redress his wound.

While taking care of his wound, I asked

him if he had another doctor's appointment this morning. The gentleman told me no, that he needed to go to the nursing home to eat breakfast with his wife.

I inquired as to her health. He told me that she had been there for a while and that she was a victim of Alzheimer's disease. As we talked, I asked if she would be upset if he was a bit late. He replied that she no longer knew who he was; she had not recognized him in five years now.

I was surprised, and asked him, "And you still go every morning, even though she doesn't know who you are?"

He smiled as he patted my hand and said, "She doesn't know me, but I still know who she is."

Such beautiful, simple love!

Duty is good. Love is superior, but duty is good. It is the catalyst that turns difficult but real love into action. It was difficult to love my mother when she had no voice for her own son, no warm smile for her son, and no loving touch for her son, me. It was difficult to love my mother when I could not even recognize her withered body, ninety percent lifeless. But that sense of duty enlivened my love so I would reach out to her, talk to her, touch her, smile at her, tell her that I love her.

And so with Penny's mom. There is a sense of duty. This is what you do—you take care of family. Mother and mother-in-law, they both deserve my love. And if, at times, when love seems reluctant or difficult and duty must be the trigger of love, that's fine.

One last remark about my own mother. I must admit that there was some guilt pushing me to make those pilgrimages to Stockton. Being raised a Catholic, I had this nagging feeling that I might be in eternal trouble if I had not gone to see Mother. When I got to the Pearly Gates, I could just see her standing behind St. Peter, urging him, "Don't let him in! He flew half way across the country four or five times a year and never came to see me! I taught him better than that. Shame on him." (Mother, dear, that's way beyond love, beyond duty—that's a good case of Catholic guilt!)

A Prayer about Duty

Lord, instill in me a sense of duty. It sounds crazy in this era of selfishness, individualism, and easy satisfaction. Duty is a lost virtue but help me get it back—at least for myself.

Duty, Lord. Your chronicles are filled with stories about duty. Cain and Abel, the fourth commandment, Joseph and his brothers, Noah and his family, Joseph, the husband of Mary—Jewish and Christian scriptures tell us again and again that we must honor our mother and father and, by extension, the rest of our family. In your eyes, Lord, family is an obligation, not a convenience. Help me to understand that and to live that.

I've agreed to take care of a very sick person in my family; a person I know is slowly dying. Or at least I've agreed that my spouse can do this. It's going to take enormous love, incredible patience, and extreme energy— both physical and emotional, and dogged perseverance. So I plead with you, Lord, as I get into this and move along on this journey, give me the grace to remember: *This is what you do for family. You take care of your family.* Remind me daily of my sense of duty and give me the strength to fulfill that obligation.

Amen.

• I Feel Helpful

As I've mentioned, I work out of our house. Such a blessing to be spared the nerve-twisting hassle of driving back and forth to work every day. Literally, I thank God for this blessing more than once a week. When we moved into this house, we took the master-on-the-main, gutted it, and transformed it into a beautiful, spacious, comfortable, and fully professional office.

Much of my day is spent there on the phone with clients, writing marketing plans, and talking with my creative director. But also, on most days I would contribute my share of housework, mostly after normal work hours, but even at times in the middle of the day. Admittedly, this was often a break from the computer more than it was a purely altruistic effort to share the house chores with Penny.

When Mom came to live with us and Penny suddenly had a lot of her time tied up in taking care of her mother, I found myself pitching in a little more. I more frequently made the bed, emptied the dishwasher, and switched the laundry. No hero here. No medal due. It simply became the thing to do. With Mom in residence, there was more work to be done. With more of a need to be with her mom, Penny had less time to do the old normal chores. More to be done; less time to get it done. A guy has to be pretty old-fashioned and a male chauvinist not to ramp up the help!

So I did just that. And as I examine my reaction to all that has gone on, I realize that I never regretted any of this extra helping—no regret, no resentment, no dissatisfaction of any kind. Perhaps it was because the "manly" demands of my soul were being called upon. The circumstances were demanding a provider. And if there is anything that strokes a man's ego, it is to be called upon to provide. So provide I did. I felt useful and satisfied in doing all those things we men so often leave to "the women."

I started this section of the book by discussing my feelings of resentment. Perhaps these feelings of being helpful balanced out the resentment. There was a surge in that negative feeling. But too, a surge in this positive feeling. I didn't feel good just because I did the dishes or the laundry more often. I felt good because I was helping the person I most love—my wife. I was responding to her need. I was living the words of my marriage vow that I would support her in her need. I could provide a little more time for her and lift a bit the weight of that burden she was under. It was not just the *physical* help that made me happy; it was the *spiritual* uplifting that resulted from those simple, physical efforts.

Years ago, I never dreamed that housework would make me a better person—more satisfied and more fulfilled. But the circumstances of my life offered me housework as a way of being truly helpful. And being helpful eased my troubles and comforted my soul, even in the face of Alzheimer's here in the house.

Prayer of a Caregiver's Helper

Jesus, thank you for making it clear that you bless us whether we have one, five, or ten talents. I'm certainly the minor character here, Lord. I'm merely in a supporting role, not the primary caregiver. Furthermore, I don't have the love, dedication and devotion my wife has. She gives her *self* to her mother. I merely give some of *my talents* in assistance.

I ask you first to bless my wife. Console her, just as she consoles her mother. Hold her up, just as she lifts her mother to the shower. Feed her with your strength, just as she feeds her mother breakfast. Clothe her in your love, just as she dresses her mother. Watch over her, just as she stays alert to any sign of her mother's momentary need. Soothe her soul, just as she puts her mother to bed.

I can't do enough to help my wife. So I ask you to support her. I cannot do enough to help my mother-in-law. So I ask you to help her.

Amen.

• Identify Your Own Positive Feelings

What keeps you going as a caregiver?

_____

_____

_____

_____

Is this particular feeling or value something you think about regularly?

_____

_____

_____

_____

Is it something you can strengthen by consciously focusing on it each day?

_____

_____

_____

_____

What other positive feelings help you cope with the difficulties of being a constant caregiver?

_____

_____

_____

_____

Are there any positive feelings or virtues that you would like to develop?

_____

_____

_____

_____

How will you develop and nourish this sought-after virtue?

_____

_____

_____

_____

By getting a book and reading about it? Finding articles about it on the internet? Talking with your best friend about it?

_____

_____

_____

_____

What will you do regularly to keep your positive feelings strong as you continue on your journey as a caregiver?

_____

_____

_____

_____

What I Have Observed

• •

No one suddenly shows the signs of having Alzheimer's in a single day. So too, no one in a single day comes to realize that a loved one has Alzheimer's. It is a gradual awareness, built mostly upon observing three key signs: forgetfulness, indifference, and physical deterioration.

• Change

My mother-in-law used to laugh a lot. She had a good sense of humor, always loved a party, and would be up dancing at the first note of an upbeat song. She would get all the girls up in a chorus line to sing and dance. Her favorite two songs were "Oh, That Nasty Man," and "Hukilau." She would just grab her daughter, her granddaughters, and her great granddaughters, line them up next to her, and start singing. After the first few words, they were all into the ritual with ample smiles, laughter, and giggling, the words mumbled, the steps stumbled, and the gestures in disarray. But by the second verse, she had them all in synch, singing lustily in perfectly choreographed steps and gestures. That was Mom. The life of the party.

And suddenly one day, she didn't know the words to "Oh That Nasty Man." What happened?

A few weeks later at another family party, she did remember the words and was up leading the family chorus line! The next time, however, she remembered some of the words, but couldn't get up to dance with her girls. What was happening?

This was the first real sign of major change—at least the first time I really noticed anything major. Now that I was noticing, change was at the same time both gradual and pervasive. Her memory didn't totally disappear one day. Like all the other changes, it was gradual. But it wasn't just her memory that was changing or declining. Everything seemed to be different: the way she looked, her hair and makeup, her carriage, her gestures, her appetite, her smiles, her conversation, the look in her eyes, the engagement with others, even the relationship with her dog. Pervasive change. Gradual, but persistent. And it was all headed in a downward direction.

Mom had been the picture of manners and politeness. "Always say thank you," she would admonish her children. "When you stand up to leave the dinner table at home, you push your chair in and fold your napkin." "There are always others, so be thoughtful and helpful." When she came to visit us several times a year after we first got married, she practiced her own admonitions, a good teacher and an excellent model to our children.

Then she came for a visit that one pivotal year. She sat down for dinner, never said "Thank you," got up from the table when she was finished, just dumped her napkin there, and left her chair pushed out like it was hastily abandoned. What was happening?

You see the picture, the pattern. Unbelievable changes in a person you know. Habits, values, abilities—everything seems to change about the person who has Alzheimer's.

• Forgetting

Alzheimer's began slowly stealing Mom's memory— occasionally, selectively, seductively, certainly. Forgetting the words to a song or the steps of a dance can be frustrating. But it is evil and cruel that Alzheimer's will make you forget the names of your own children or the name of your beloved, deceased husband. Mom got to the point where she did not know what day it was, what she did that day, or what she ate for dinner an hour ago. We know that Alzheimer's attacks the brain. Obviously, it enjoys attacking memory!

Many of the disease's early signs, taken individually, can be attributed to simple old age. One is tired after many years of trying to make everyone happy. So one just stops trying so hard, gives in to aching bones and tired spirits, becomes slower, less enthusiastic, a little more withdrawn. But when your parent or spouse has such a wholesale loss of cherished memories, realize that Alzheimer's has arrived. Expect things to get worse.

From my observations—of my own mother, my sister, and my mother-in-law, this memory loss, both deep and wide, is a sure sign of Alzheimer's.

• Indifference

My mother-in-law led a magical and blessed life thanks to her husband. Pop loved her with abundance of love and worldly goods. Mom enjoyed life, savored its goods, and participated in its daily blessings. She enjoyed shopping, enjoyed her children, and enjoyed her friends. Basically she was thoughtful, kind, and generous to family and friends. And she was always ready for a party.

But then we started to see her pulling away. It was gradual but real. My wife would ask, "Mom, do you want to go look for a new dress?"

"No. Not really."

"Mom, let's call Louise (her best friend of fifty-plus years). She'd love to hear from you."

"No. I don't want to talk."

And so it went with increasing frequency. A one time connected woman becoming more and more indifferent to her friends and the things she used to enjoy. At first, I used to think these were responses of a woman who was simply tired. She just didn't feel up to shopping or staying on the phone for what could be a long time. We all have moments like this and, God knows, we don't have to be old! All we need is to be tired.

But the attitude continued, appeared with increasing

frequency, soon became a pattern, and then established itself as the norm. Here again was that gradual but relentless insistency of Alzheimer's. Everything about it starts slowly, subtly, almost sneakily. But once it is there, once it starts, it never goes away. It feeds on its victim like an alien monster that cannot be killed. It grows, devours more of its unwilling host, becomes stronger and more vicious, and constantly envelops an entire body and soul until the old, tired, sick person just gives up—probably without even realizing it!

Evil, penetrating, permeating Alzheimer's gradually extinguishes the spark and light of the soul. What remains is a person without spunk—an indifferent person.

• Physical Deterioration

Every elderly person deteriorates, some more or faster than others. There are the well-documented stooped women with osteoporosis, the old men with prostate cancer, and the hundreds of others with a million ailments that diminish our human bodies. Cancers of almost any part of the body, diseases of the heart, failings of the entire immune system, imbalances of the endocrine system and more. We are partly physical. We deteriorate.

But with Alzheimer's, there is a more than normal deterioration. I've been involved with sick people since 1961. My observation has been that most "old age" sickness can be pinpointed to cardio problems, endocrine imbalance, malfunctions of the immune system, and other specific areas. But in these recent years of observing Alzheimer's, I notice a shut-down of many bodily systems. There is no obvious, sound-the-alarm problem with the heart, the lungs, the liver or kidneys, the sense of balance. There just is suddenly the recognition of a general deterioration of the body. It doesn't *happen* suddenly. But one day you just *notice:* She has really slowed down! It was a gradual change, looking back. But you realize that your *awareness* of that gradual deterioration was sudden.

If your dad gets a heart attack, both the attack and your awareness of it are instant. If your ninety-year-old mom falls and breaks her hip, fact and awareness are quick, immediate. The terrible thing about Alzheimer's is that it is sneaky. It creeps up on its victim. If that victim is your loved one—your mother or father or spouse—it creeps up on you!

A Prayer of Thanksgiving

Thank you, Lord, for this earthly, physical life.

Thank you for my five senses. Thank you for the gift of sight, to see the promise of the sun, the giving of the flowers, the smiles of a child. Thank you for the gift of hearing, to hear the drum roll of the thunder, the songs of the birds, and the symphony of Beethoven. Thank you for the gift of touch, to feel the slide of silk, the strength of steel, and the softness of marshmallows. Thank you for the gift of smell, to appreciate fine perfume, gardenias, and vanilla. Thank you for the gift of taste, to savor chocolate cake, fettuccini, and a smooth merlot.

Thank you for my brain, for balance, for motion. Thank you for dreams, desires, and determination. Thank you for independence. Thank you for all these good things that contribute to my life today. I realize that some day I too may lose them all. But while I possess them, I am grateful for them. Normally I take them for granted. But today, as I look at this patient I see dying each day, I realize what wonderful gifts they are. And I say thank you.

Amen.

The Worst Part

● ●

For you, the caregiver or spouse of the caregiver, the worst part of Alzheimer's in your house is not the physical disease. It is the fact that it demands daily presence and work on your part. The daily-ness of it is what will get to you. And the "little things" will bother you much more than the major problems.

• The Daily-ness of It All

The worst part of having Alzheimer's in your home is not the sickness itself or any specific manifestation of the disease. You've heard enough about Alzheimer's even if you just half-heartedly listened to several of the hundred reports on the daily news. You've heard about the change at the very core of a person who becomes struck by this hideous sickness. You've heard about the forgetfulness, the wandering of mind and sometimes body; the loss of awareness, the lack of interest, the shut down. You've heard about the incontinence, the Depends, and the need for constant physical care. In general, you know the symptoms. Probably at least six of your friends have a relative suffering from Alzheimer's. If you start to ask, you'll probably find at least two or three acquaintances that are actually caring for a parent with Alzheimer's!

If Alzheimer's comes to your home, the worst thing about it will be the daily-ness of it. Alzheimer's never gives up. The symptoms never go away. Likewise, the need for care never goes away. If Alzheimer's comes to your home, you will have to deal with it every single day. There is no vacation, no weekend break, no holiday. It is constant in its grasp of your loved one. Therefore, your election to be caregiver is a choice to deal with this constantly.

Anyone can rise to the need of taking care of a sick parent. But it takes courage, endurance, constancy, perseverance, and heroism to commit to daily care without ceasing or any end in sight. We can all care for an hour, for an occasion, or even for a year or two. But to care daily—every single day, for a long, open-ended time is true heroism. It is exactly this daily caring that Alzheimer's demands. It not only takes the life of its immediate victim. It also demands much of the life of whoever chooses to care for its victim!

To change your mom's Depend is a nuisance; to do it every single day is a hardship.

To shower your mom is a nuisance; to do it every single day is a hardship.

To brush your mom's teeth is a nuisance; to do it every single day is a hardship.

To dress your mom is a nuisance; to do it every single day is a hardship.

To feed your mom three meals is a nuisance; to do it every single day is a hardship.

To clean up after your mom is a nuisance; to do it every single day is a hardship.

To see your mom decline is always difficult; to watch it every day is a hardship.

When I went to work after post-graduate school, I quickly saw the blessing of variety. I vowed not to be in a rut, having a single job to do every day. I sought and found variety. Recognizing the kaleidoscopic aspect of life, I cherished a degree of complexity in my life. I did not want everything to be blue or red or magenta. I wanted to see them all, whether sequentially planned or randomly chaotic.

To a great degree I've been able to live this aspect of my life dream. But I notice that my wife does not have this luxury at this time in her life. As the primary caregiver to her mother, Penny is caught in a single-focus life. From when she gets up in the morning until she goes to sleep at night, the care of her mother is her single focus. She can be shopping or catching a rare and quick lunch with a good friend, but always on her mind is her mother and what she must do for her. It is the daily-ness of the disease that exacts from the caregiver a constant and daily focus of concern, worry, caring, and serving.

Even when she goes to sleep, my wife is burdened with the thoughts and worries of her mother's care. A baby-monitor sits on the night table next to her bed, ready to alarm her if Mom gets up in the middle of the night and falls or tries to wander off.

Every single day. Every single night.

The Prayer of St. Francis

Lord, make me an instrument of your peace.
Where there is hatred, let me sow love;
Where there is injury, pardon;
Where there is doubt, faith;
Where there is despair, hope;
Where there is darkness, light;
And where there is sadness, joy.

O Divine Master, grant that I may not so much seek
to be consoled as to console;
to be understood as to understand;
to be loved as to love.
For it is in giving that we receive;
It is in pardoning that we are pardoned;
And it is in dying that we are born to eternal life.

Amen

(Copied from a hand written paper in my mother's prayer book.)

The Little Things

We all like our own way of doing things. It's the way we were raised. Not necessarily right or wrong. But it is what we see as the norm, the preferable. Each of us grows up with customs and rules taught by our experiences— some forever ingrained from childhood, some learned later in life. Somehow we let our emotions get attached to these learned ways of how daily life ought to be. There are things based on the big values—respect for women, honoring parents, being polite. Other values are strong but of less importance—table manners, making ones bed every day, expressing gratitude. And some are truly arbitrary but nonetheless important—how to put dishes in the dishwasher, driving habits, rolling up the toothpaste tube. As we were raised, so we envision what is correct and proper for all of these whether they reflect truly important values or simply arbitrary custom.

When we get married, we learn to adjust our sense of "the right way." If we can't adjust, give in a bit, give and take, or compromise—at least when essential values are not at stake—we probably will have a failed marriage. A husband and wife find ways to adjust in order to get along amicably or peacefully. This compromising is not really difficult. We just do it once we realize the need because we love each other and *want* to find agreement. If I was raised putting all the knives in one section of the dishwasher basket or all the forks in another section of the basket, I readily adjust to seeing forks and knives mixed because that's the way my wife has always done it. As long as they all come out clean, what do I care if she prefers it another way? I'm married. Therefore I adjust. And I am happy to adjust—especially in the little things.

This is not so with Alzheimer's in your home.

It will be those little things that kill you.

Deep within my soul I can accept that there is an extra person living in my house, a person who demands a lot of attention. I can accept that this person draws a lot of my wife's attention away from me to her. I can accept that mine and Penny's "us time"—our time shared together as just the two of us, experiencing and enjoying something together exclusively—is much less than I had planned for years ago. I can accept the time dedicated to caring for Mom—hours each morning and throughout the day. I can even accept the TV blasting loudly all afternoon and evening.

It's the little things I can't stand. I choose not to want to accept them. I choose to let them bother me. This sort of choice makes no sense; it is not commendable. It is an acknowledged flaw that I allow to continue. (Why? I realize it is childish, irrational, and a stress of my own making.)

I let it disturb me that Mom never says "Thank you"

to my wife, who cooks her meals for her. I let it disturb me that Mom never pushes her chair in when she gets up from the dinner table. I get upset when every single night she leaves her used paper napkin and two or three Kleenexes at her place and walks away from the dinner table. I get mad that she never pushes the "off" button on the phone after she speaks to her son in Las Vegas. I get peeved when she routinely leaves a gum wrapper on the floor of the car.

These things are not important at all. I know that. Yet, I let them bother me. The poor woman probably has no recognition that she even does these things. She's losing her mind! Alzheimer's is eroding her recognition, awareness, and comprehension much as the sun slowly, relentlessly, and certainly fades the vibrant colors of an advertisement painted on a country barn-side.

Life is filled with choices. We choose to let some differences bother us while accepting others. I find that the little things get to me. Perhaps it is because we prepare for battle and are ready for the more serious onslaughts. Fine. I just suggest that you prepare more thoroughly if Alzheimer's comes to your house. Prepare for the big difficulties. But also prepare for the little things.

A Buddhist Prayer for Peace

May all beings everywhere plagued with sufferings of body and mind quickly be freed from their illnesses.

May those frightened cease to be afraid,
And may those bound be free.
May the powerless find power,
And may people think of befriending one another.
May those who find themselves in trackless, fearful
wilderness ~the children, the aged, the unprotected ~be
guarded by beneficial celestials.

(Author unknown)

How I Cope

● ●

Dictionary.com defines "cope" in this way:
—*verb (used without object)*

> 1. to struggle or deal, esp. on fairly even terms or with some degree of success (usually fol. by *with*): *I will try to cope with his rudeness.*

> 2. to face and deal with responsibilities, problems, or difficulties, esp. successfully or in a calm or adequate manner: *After his breakdown he couldn't cope any longer.*

To my way of thinking, the operative words in these definitions of "cope" are "struggle" and "difficulty." (Although the word "breakdown" did get my attention!) The difficulties are the starting point. One does not cope with the easy things of life. No one struggles with the pleasant, the fun, and the easy-going. I need to share with you my tools for coping precisely because when Alzheimer's comes you *will* be in a *difficult* situation and you *will* have to *deal* with it.

I've already stated the difficulties that Alzheimer's will bring to you when it comes to your house in the body of your mother or father. There is shock when you realize how sick he or she really is. There is worry because you don't comprehend what is going to happen. There are huge emotional burdens (See "How I Feel.") There are financial burdens, from medical bills and professional help all the way down to higher food and utility bills. There is the problem of intrusion with an attendant loss to varying degrees of your own privacy, your own space, and your own sense of normalcy. There is additional shopping, cooking, feeding, and clean up. To be honest about Alzheimer's in your house, you must recognize that there will be difficulties, problems, and struggles. And you'll have to cope with them.

• I Balance

So how have I coped so far? One answer (there are many) is found within that second definition I quoted earlier: "to face and deal with responsibilities, problems. ..." Exactly. I cope by facing and dealing with both the responsibilities and the problems. If I focus on just the problems, I will become negative and bitter. But if I balance the problems with a sense of responsibility, then I can cope. Penny and I constantly respond to people who ask how we do it with this simple statement: "This is what you do for your family." Mom is family. So we take care of her because she needs taking care of. This fundamental sense of family and a sense of responsibility to family get me through many a day of Mom's sickness.

A sense of responsibility is just one tool for coping. Another attitude, which I believe to be essential, is admitting. I admit that this sick woman coming to live in my house is a problem. For some strange reason, the word "problem" has disappeared from modern speech. Perhaps it is because people don't like to face difficulties, so they don't even accept the word "problem." Now we seem to have nothing but issues. Well, dealing with Alzheimer's is much bigger than a mere *issue*. Believe me. It is a *Problem*. With a capital "P."

You will not cope with Alzheimer's in your home if you do not see it as a problem on one hand, and balance it with a sense of responsibility on the other.

A Prayer for Courage

Lord, I've always been told that I would never be saddled with more than I can handle. Well, thank you for that assurance. In my mind I can believe it, but in my heart I'm worried. My patient can live for years with this disease. And the caring must be day after day after day. Alzheimer's doesn't take the weekend off or take a vacation. I'm scared. I'm afraid I may not have the perseverance to continue this caregiving for years. Just the thought of doing this every single day for years is daunting.

How am I going to feed her every day, for years?

How am I going to bathe her, every single day?

How am I going to dress her, every single day?
Actually doing this each day is not the problem.
It's the very *thought* of having to do this that scares me.
Give me courage, Lord.

How will I talk to her distorted mind every single day?

How will I smile at her unresponsive face every single day?

How will I say, "I love you," when the words are never returned?

Actually doing this each day is not the problem.

It's the very *thought* of having to do this that scares me.

Give me courage, Lord.

Give me courage.

Amen.

• I Admit

Next you will need to admit your feelings. At first, I felt guilty about feeling resentment. Certainly I did not want to tell my wife I resented her mother—no matter what the reason. From this point of view (and only this point of view) it would be easier if the sick woman were *my* mother, not Penny's. But when I finally admitted that I felt all this resentment and had the courage to verbalize it to my wife, I did feel a level of freedom. This was coping—to admit my feelings, face them, and deal with them. It will be impossible to cope with your feelings if you do not first admit them.

The next step for me in coping with the stressful, terrible situation in my house was to admit my shortcomings. Once I was able to admit (a difficult thing for me, who is perfect) that I was not the most caring, wonderful, self-giving, altruistic, sacrificing, noble, generous, magnanimous person on earth, I could deal a little better with the situation and my response to it. Coping comes only after an admission of imperfection. God doesn't have to cope because he is perfect and can understand all, put everything in perspective, and deal with everything with absolute power and love. But I need to find another way—which I won't even look for until I admit that I am not God!

A Prayer for Honesty

Lord, you once said that we should let our speech be, "Yes. Yes." And "No. No." If you meant that literally, I've failed you miserably!

Perhaps you were admonishing us to be honest. Because of my own inadequacies, worries, and insufficient trust of others, I often neglect to speak up. Sometimes I ignore the truth or shade it. Help me, first, to be honest with my own feelings and admit the most inner truths about myself.

Give me the courage to discuss my feelings honestly but sensitively with my spouse. Guide me not to complain, but simply to share my self. Make me humble enough to trust my spouse to accept me as I truly am, no matter our differences of thought or feeling. Make me meek that I might accept my lover's responses, be they accepting, admonishing, or challenging. Give me the grace to grow in honesty through these intimate discussions with my spouse.

Just speaking openly about this difficult problem of Alzheimer's and caregiving can mold a more honest appraisal of the situation and a more honest approach to dealing with it. I need that honesty, Lord, in order to cope better with life today.

Amen.

• I Pray

My next coping skill is prayer. I believe it to be a blessing that I happened to be raised in a devout Catholic family. I was taught to pray from childhood. Prayer has always been an integral part of my life. It keeps me in daily touch with the three "big" virtues: faith, hope, and love. (Sometimes I believe that the greatest of these is not love but hope!) Prayer keeps life in perspective. Every single morning, I can sit in some quiet spot and start the day by thanking God for the good and beautiful he has placed in my life. I thank him for the treasures of the universe, for my wife, my family, my brains, for the ability to cope, for the gift of choice, for the examples of love, for health, and for the means to help my wife, whom I truly love, take care of her slowly dying mother. In prayer, I ask God to forgive my pettiness and grant me the courage to deal positively with a negative situation. Prayer is a spiritual multi-vitamin that each day strengthens my soul and brings courage to my decisions. Prayer, for me, is essential to coping.

The Lord's Prayer

Our Father, who art in heaven,
hallowed be thy name.
Thy Kingdom come,
thy will be done,
on earth as it is in heaven.
Give us this day our daily bread.
And forgive us our trespasses,
as we forgive those who trespass against us.
And lead us not into temptation,
but deliver us from evil.
For thine is the kingdom, the power and the glory, for ever and ever.

Amen

(Written from my memory and my heart)

• I Escape

Fortunately, circumstances are such that I can escape from the immediate environment regularly. I recognize that it is very difficult for some to "get away" from Alzheimer's and its grip on the caregiver. I think of my brother-in-law. He alone cares for my sister in a two-bedroom apartment in Oakland. It is a small space, and he is with her virtually 24/7. He has precious few opportunities to take a break from the constant, unceasing tasks of caring for his Alzheimer's wife. I admire him and admit that I'm not sure I could live up to his gracious and dedicated level of caring. Just to be *present all the time,* as he is, amazes me. He has to stay with her because he has not set up a network of help that can relieve him.

Find a way to get help. And the help I'm talking about is getting some person to come in so you can go out. You have to get away and take a break. You need to reset your perspectives, rekindle your appreciations, and recharge your soul. Step out of the house so you can step back in and step up to the challenges.

I try to get away every other day that Mom is with us. I'll go to the local LA Fitness or go take a swim. I'll go to a men's discussion group every week. What we discuss is not important, but every week I get my mind out of the house and hear something new and valuable at these meetings. Some days, I'll drive seven or eight minutes to the bookstore and stay only ten minutes without being serious about buying a book. I'm escaping. A new book I do not need. To get away for a half hour—this I need.

Perhaps, I recently realized, I just go somewhere to remind myself that I can. Alzheimer's is jail. It is shackles. It is the ultimate grip that robs one of free movement. While rubbing shoulders with this jailer, I want to express vividly that it has no hold on me. I can go where I want. I can escape. Therefore, I do escape.

Some may see this as running as opposed to coping. I see it as coping, in that I balance my recognition of Mom's plight with the recognition that I am still free. Alzheimer's is evil. But it is not universal. The goodness of life remains despite the evil within it. You need to think this way in order to cope. You need to enjoy life as fully as you can, move as freely as you can, laugh as much as you can and, always, think as positively as you can.

A Prayer for Rest

God, even you took a day off after six days of creating a wonderful world! Give me some rest here. I'm trying to create a better world for Mom and my wife. It has been more than six days and appears that it will go on forever! Certainly I am not stronger than you. Do not test my endurance. Give me a break.

Jesus, for all his wisdom and power, escaped from time to time to refresh himself and restore his focus. Can I not have the same respite? At times, there seems to be no relief. The attention, focusing, and giving are constant.

Let me know that it is okay to take a little time for me.
Let me know that I can take time for me without guilt.
Let me know that some time for me is good, important.
Give me the creativity to find my times for true rest.

Give me the faith to believe that you will take care while I rest.

Amen.

• I Affirm

Many years ago, I learned about a mental process called "affirmations." Simply put, affirmations are positive self-talks stated in the present tense. The wonder of affirmations is that these positive thoughts, regularly repeated and imagined, do build a positive spirit. I thoroughly believe in affirmations, believe they positively affect my daily outlook on life, and believe they enable me to cope with the difficulties that Mom's sickness has brought to our home.

This is not the place to defend or to teach a class on affirmations. But I can share a few of the ones I repeat each day.

- I am really happy being the unique and very special person that I am.

- I have unconditional warm regards for all people at all times.

- I show that I am 100 percent alive by thinking, speaking, and acting with great enthusiasm.

- I easily relax as deeply as I wish at any time.

- I am completely healthy in mind and body at all times.

- I face all my problems with great courage and thus cope with them positively and successfully.

- I have ample leisure without guilt.

- This day, I enjoy taking care of my patient.

I believe these statements help get me through the crisis in my home. I repeat them every day no matter what is going on. As they are seen, spoken, and heard within my own head, they become more and more the reality of my life. They become the reality not by magic, but because I slowly and eventually *make* them happen. My mind builds my future. If I keep thinking negative thoughts, my daily life will become more and more negative. If, on the other hand, I keep thinking positive thoughts, I will create a more and more positive daily existence for myself. I believe this. It works for me. Affirmations are one of my specific, deliberate, effective coping tools.

A Prayer of Responsibility

There is a conflict in my heart, Lord. Sometimes I think I should just leave everything up to you. You told me to have faith that you would care for me. I've been taught to pray, "Thy will be done."

On the other hand, I have read the gospel of the talents and saw how you got angry at the man who didn't get aggressive and use his God-given talents to better his own life.

So, do I leave it all to you, your wisdom, and your power? Or do I take charge of my own life? Perhaps a little of both? Then, where is the balance?

I see the answer in the book of Genesis, Lord, in the story of Creation. No matter what else there is to learn, one truth stands strong, undeniable, and infallible: You made me in your own image and likeness. I am, therefore, a creator—a creator of my own living. You initiated life in me, but handed me the responsibility to make of myself what I can, to use the talents you gave me to fashion my person. You gave me the power to become what I want, as I want.

In gratitude and humility, I strive every day to make myself a better person. I dictate not every circumstance of my life, but certainly I can dictate my response to every circumstance. I can dictate my response to this sickness, to this decision to have Mom live with us, and to the daily difficulties of caring for her. The choice is mine. Day by day, I can choose to become more patient or more resentful this day.

Please give me the grace to choose patience. Just for today. Tomorrow I will have another opportunity to choose. And we'll talk again then.

Amen.

• I Focus

I cope with my sick mother-in-law living in my house by focusing on the love I have for my wife. When I married Penny, I promised her I would do everything

I could to be the best husband. More important than providing tangible things is my daily choice to support her, encourage her, and help her. It is so difficult for my wife to take care of her Alzheimer's-gripped mother. My wedding day promise from over thirty years ago must be realized today if it is not to be mere empty words. That promise to do everything I could helps me now to step up and stand side by side with her.

There are days when I wish my mother-in-law would just go away. Literally. Go away to God, go away to live with one of her sons forever, go away to a nursing home. Just go away, out of my home. No! Out of my life. And spare my wife the incessant, insistent demands of caring for an Alzheimer's parent.

But Penny has chosen, for her own noble and blessed reasons, to take care of her mother. And my love for this caring, giving woman encourages and enables me to be a real part of the caregiving. Every day, my love for my wife moves me to gladly offer another day of dealing with the sickness. It is not, I admit, 100 percent enthusiastic, but it is not completely reluctant either. There may be reluctant moments in any given day, but the overall attitude, the mental/emotional posture is positive. I want to help my wife. I choose to support her this day. I want to assist her with her chores of caregiving today. Love must take forms of action in the human being. My love for my wife morphs into deeds. My focus on my wife and my love for her help me cope with Alzheimer's in our home.

A Prayer for My Wife

Lord, bless my wife.

She is already abundantly blessed, full of your grace.
But she needs strength, for the day is long.
Bless her, Lord.

She is so smart, full of intelligence and common sense.
But she needs strength, for some days make little sense.
Bless her, Lord.

She is kind, generous, and thoughtful of everyone.
But she needs strength, for we all take from her.
Bless her, Lord.

She is a living example of your love.
But she needs strength, for she is only human.
Bless her, Lord.

She gives generously, never counting the cost.
But she needs strength, for there is indeed a cost.
Bless her, Lord.

She constantly smiles and encourages others.
But she needs strength, for there are moments of sorrow.
Bless her Lord.

Bless her with your strength, your wisdom, your love,
your joy.

Amen.

• I Connect

There's a friend of mine whom I can talk to honestly when I feel overwhelmed by frustration or anger. I don't unload on him often, but whenever I do, it helps me tremendously. I don't ask for advice; he gives me none. I just talk; he just listens. For me it is therapeutic.

About once a month, I call a lady in California, a friend I have known for years. I always ask how she is—it is the apparent reason I call. After she tells me about herself and her children, she always asks me, "And how are you doing with your mom?" Usually I just say, "Fine." But often I relate a short story about some frustration, or express a concern about my wife getting no rest, or just express an exasperated wish that we need a real break from all this.

And, of course, there is the weekly phone call to JJ, my brother-in-law, who is taking care of my sister with Alzheimer's. Often nothing is said in these conversations about Alzheimer's or caregiving; sometimes it is the explicit topic of the exchange. But always, there is the implied understanding, which is its own form of support. I know that he understands my difficulties, frustrations, and moments of anger and exhaustion from the daily giving of total care. And he knows that I understand his difficulties, frustrations, and moments of anger and exhaustion from the daily giving of total care. These exchanges provide silent, secret, indescribable, but very real relief.

George, Patty, and JJ—three loving people that nurture me, revive me, and enable me.

I only realized that it is so important to connect and reach out to others when someone told me, "You know, you're not Superman. You don't have to do this all by yourself. There are plenty of people who will help you." I was reluctant to accept that push for several reasons. First, because of my stubborn pride. After all, I do have a tendency to believe I am Superman. Or perhaps it is that I am a typical Scorpio: silent, quiet, figure it out alone, be strong, don't complain, and just get it done. And there is reluctance on my part to burden others with my troubles. It's the way I was raised; it is the way I've been all my life—an independent streak.

As said, reaching out revives me, nurtures me, and enables me. Just talking with someone who has a little understanding of what I am going through removes some of the weight of the burden. Just knowing that someone else cares about this caregiver gives me extra strength. And that enables me to continue—for another day, a week, a month.

These are not counseling sessions. At times, nothing explicit is said about either Alzheimer's or caregiving. Sometimes that is all we talk about. Mostly, on the surface, it is just a conversation. But under the surface, it is a connection with someone who tries to understand how I feel about constant caregiving, a connection with someone who knows that I hurt or am frustrated or tired, and a connection with someone who is not judging me or condemning me for my worries, reluctance, anger, or exhaustion. It is not counseling, not fixing, not advising that is important here; it is the connection itself. It is therapeutic.

I must tell you about some wonderful caregivers I met recently. Four sisters, all of whom are giving care to their four brothers who have Alzheimer's. They live separately, each taking care of one of their brothers! They connect every night. They have a mini-conference-call, the four sisters talking to each other. One of them told me that she couldn't go on without these nightly calls. The best part of the conversation, she says, is when one of them starts describing some silly thing her brother did this particular day. They are able to share and to laugh. They don't give each other advice; they don't help each other with chores; they don't relieve each other for an hour or two—all they do is connect. This connecting is what nurtures them, revives them, and enables them.

A Prayer for Being Real

I'm not alone.
So why don't I reach out for help?

What are my excuses?
Too busy? Embarrassed? Afraid to be a burden on anyone?

I need to get out of my self-pity, to reach out to others, to ask for help.
I need to acknowledge that I need help.

I need to *ask* for that help, since it will not come on its own.
I need to get real about the enormity of my needs and the limits of my abilities.
I need to pick up the phone and admit to someone that I need help.
I need to call a friend and ask for an hour's help.
I need to ask a friend, or a neighbor, to "baby-sit" so I can get a break.
I need to call the Alzheimer's Association and be open with them.
I need to let someone know my needs, if not my feelings.

I'm not alone.
God give me the wisdom to go asking.
For I *will* receive.

• I Laugh

There is a lot to laugh about when you live with an Alzheimer's patient. Because their brain does not function correctly, they make mistakes of speech, judgment, and response. There is humor in some of those mistakes.

Some would immediately criticize even the thought of laughing at an Alzheimer's patient. Okay. So you don't laugh *at* the patient, but be ready to laugh *about* what the patient does.

The unexpected is a classic source of humor. Mom awakes at three o'clock in the morning, dresses herself, grabs an empty suitcase, and, fortunately, gets caught before she can open the front door. Penny, just roused from sleep, asks, "What are you doing, Mom?" "I'm going home." Penny replies, "You *are* home!"

Now we could get aggravated over this or even angry for being awakened in the middle of the night. Or we can go back to bed and laugh about it for a minute or two before falling back to sleep. A ninety-four year old lady with an empty suitcase walking down the street at three in the morning. Certainly Leno or Letterman could do something with this scene. We tried to and fell asleep.

One morning, I asked Mom if she wanted a cup of coffee. Yes. When I bring the coffee to her room, she is holding an envelope and asked me what I had in my hand. I told her it was her coffee. "This is my coffee," she said waving the envelope. I did not ask, did not argue, and did not even try to understand what she might be thinking. But the thought of her sipping hot coffee out of an envelope did bring a little smile to my lips.

In every situation, you have a choice as to how you react. Always try to react by finding a little humor in the unexpected things your patient will say or do (or try to do).

To stimulate her mind, I tried one day to engage Mom in a game of scrabble. We each had our letters in our racks. I had to get up to answer the phone. When I came back to the table, she had carefully replaced her tiles with peanuts. It struck me as funny, wondering what she could spell with seven peanuts.

Another way I try to inject humor into the

Alzheimer's environment is by telling Mom the oldest, corniest jokes I can think of at any moment. At first, I thought I was doing this for her–a little light, momentary entertainment. But eventually I realized that I was doing this as much for me as for her. There is enough stress and frustration that comes automatically each day. I find attempts at humor, even silly humor, relieve some of that emotional tension.

A Prayer of Laughter

God, do you laugh at our silliness?

Do you sit around and laugh when we spend so much venom and anger arguing over whether or not you created the world? You either just created it or set it up to evolve. So why argue about it? You must think we are silly.

Do you laugh when I ask you to help me win the lottery but forget to buy a ticket?

Do you laugh a little at me when I pray for my team to win because you know that the other team is sending up just as many prayers?

Were you having a little fun when you created the panda?

Maybe when you created me! Well, that's okay. Help me not to take myself all so seriously.

And help me to see humor wherever it is, especially when it's staring me in the face—or *is* my face!

Amen.

Your Personal Plan for Coping

Write down your answers to the following questions. Write down your own plans for coping with the difficulties of caregiving.

What do you do now to help you make it through the day without feeling overwhelmed and exhausted?

_____

_____

_____

_____

Are you at the stage of fighting every unpleasant and difficult reality? Or can you at least admit that what is, is? Once you admit what is real, you have a chance of embracing and dealing with it in a healthy and positive way. What do you need to come to grips with? Take five minutes right now to think about it and start dealing with it.

_____

_____

_____

_____

My plan:

And come back tomorrow to think about it for another five minutes.

_____

_____

_____

_____

My plan:

If you see even the smallest ember of faith glowing in your soul, do you pray? Might prayer and the recognition of a higher power help you cope with the details of your own life? Do you want to pray? Do you prefer reading prayers from a book or would you rather just speak spontaneously to God from the depths of your soul? If you choose to pray, when is the best time of the day to do that?

_____

_____

_____

_____

My plan:

When can you take five minutes to read your affirmations? As soon as you wake up, even before you get out of bed? Right after your first cup of coffee? Immediately before you go to sleep at night?

_____

_____

_____

_____

My plan:

You need a life-line, someone to converse with on a fairly regular basis. It might be a relative, a friend, or a neighbor. Tell a friend that you need someone to talk to, even if it is just over the phone. Make a list of those people you can ask to call regularly.

_____

_____

_____

_____

My plan:

Create for yourself a chance to escape. Try to find someone to come to your home regularly to sit with your sick one while you leave the house for at least an hour. If you cannot think of anyone to ask or find anyone who will help, call the local Alzheimer's Association office, your church, or your local community center. It might take a little work to find them, but there are people who will help you.

_____

_____

_____

_____

My plan:

Identify something beautiful or inspiring in your house that you can focus on every single day. As a caregiver you focus daily on sickness, if not an accelerated process of death. It is important to compensate that with something or someone emotionally inspiring.

_____

_____

_____

_____

My plan:

A good way to find humor in your daily life is to keep a journal. Each evening, think back over the events of the day and try to identify one saying or action that had a humorous aspect to it. Focus on that moment of humor and capture it in writing. As you write in your journal it will become more prominent in your memory. That little humor of today might be just what you need to help you deal with tomorrow.

_____

_____

_____

_____

My plan:

What other mechanisms—thoughts, words, or deeds—can you think of to help you cope with the daily difficulties of caregiving?

_____

_____

_____

_____

My plan:

_____

_____

_____

_____

Teasing

●●●●●●●●●●●●●●●●●●●●●●●●●●●

There come, irregularly but certainly, hours or full days when Mom is alert, communicative (as opposed to merely talkative) energetic, pleasant, and even fun. Where does this come from? Sometimes I think she must have hit her head and snapped all those synapses back into connection and function!

• Those Days of Returning Lucidity

Our good friends have known for years that we are taking care of Mom. But on certain days, if they didn't know better, they would think there is nothing wrong with this woman. On occasion, she can seem as ordinary as any elderly woman in reasonably good health. She is alert and engaging. This is some sinister proof that we cannot really understand or control Alzheimer's. One day I think her mind is completely gone; the next, I am confronted with someone who is just a little slow but apparently lucid.

These moments are true gifts. These are the moments when my wife can enjoy her mom again, as a bonus. It is filial overtime—an extra quarter. It is as if they were given a second chance to communicate again—positively, enthusiastically. These moments are sporadic, without advanced notification, and irregular in duration. But they are wonderful when they come and while they last.

One day we were at a friend's house for dinner. We brought Mom with us. As we were getting ready to leave, Mom spied a piano in the living room, shuffled over, pulled out the bench, sat down, and proceeded to play a few tunes. She was good! This woman had not played the piano in the last twenty years. In the last six years, I would have judged her totally incapable of playing the scale. Yet here comes this moment, a sort of reincarnation, a resurrection of some musical spirit and physical gift that had succumbed to Alzheimer's.

Then, as quickly as it appeared, the talent or the gift disappears again into the foggy nowhere of Alzheimer's.

I must admit that I am more excited for Penny during these times than I am for Mom. I have no idea of the comprehension levels in Mom's brain on an ordinary day or on one of these "return" days. I see it as perhaps a little bit of teasing...Here! Have your mind back for a while. Then it is ripped out again by Alzheimer's. But for my wife, it is a time to reconnect, to enjoy again the pleasures of an earlier day, and to express again her love and gratefulness to her mother. She sees it as an added wonderful moment in their relationship, another chance to enjoy the precious woman who gave her life, and another moment to thank her.

I feel tremendous gratitude on these occasions. It is so nice to see Mom so alert and my wife so happy. These days give you a break from all those negative feelings. They give you something positive to dwell on for a day. They remind you that in the bitter snows of winter lies a seed that becomes a rose.

A Prayer of Humility

I guess we're not really in charge of things, Lord. Certainly not the master plan. I like to think that I am in charge of everything in my circle of life. But here is a disease I know little about; a sickness that can throw my daily routines into a spin.

I don't want to be a wimp, Lord, leaving everything to you or blaming you for everything that goes bad in my life. I want to use the talents you've given me and take honest responsibility for my actions and my life. But let me understand my limits. All creation is bigger than me. Nature is stronger than me. A tiny tick can kill me. An unseen virus can wipe out good health. An ocean wave can literally snap my body in two. Yes, I am powerful, but not almighty. Yes, I am intelligent, but not omniscient.

Lord, help me to balance my pride in how wonderful you have made me and my humility in recognizing how much I am at the mercy of the forces of your universe. Perhaps there is incentive for me to grow in the very recognition that I am only one small part of your creation.

Help me to grow, Lord, to be a better person, to be better caregiver, and to be a better steward of your creation.

Amen.

What I Fear

●●●●●●●●●●●●●●●●●●●●●●●●

It is said that we fear the unknown. But I believe that, to some degree, we fear the known. If I did not know Alzheimer's through observing my mother, my sister, and my mother-in-law, I would not fear it. But what I observe does frighten me because I know that I could develop this dreadful disease.

• Losing My Freedom, Dignity, and Pride

So you know how I feel, and you know how I cope. I'm sure any psychiatrist who has read my words to this point already knows my fears. He or she could write an enlightening chapter, based solely on what I've already committed to print. So I might as well be honest and blunt about my fears.

I do not fear getting old. By some people's count, I already am.

I fear getting feeble.

I fear getting senile.

I fear getting Alzheimer's.

I fear losing my freedom.

I fear losing my mind.

I fear being unable to come and go as I please.

I fear needing someone to dress me the rest of my life.

I fear someone having to put clean Depends on me each day.

I fear not having a conscious purpose.

I fear doing nothing until someone tells me to do it.

I fear doing nothing on my own; nothing without a caregiver.

As I think about this list, as I write it, I come to the awareness that, bottom line, I fear not having any pride. "Pride goeth before the fall." Well, this fall (succumbing to Alzheimer's) will certainly take away any and all pride I have today. As I witness Alzheimer's in my home today, as I have witnessed it in my sister and my mother, I believe that Alzheimer's gets to the stage where it leaves its victim totally bereft of pride. I fear being without pride.

I fear this, and all the obvious steps leading up to it (enumerated above) probably because I am too proud. Perhaps I need to start learning more about humility.

When I was about twenty-five years old, my work often brought me to many hospitals and nursing homes. One of the hospitals I visited regularly had one of the busiest ER rooms in California. Kaiser Hospital had contracts with the city, the county, and the state to pick up every emergency in the area—from auto wrecks to fires to suicides to murders. I saw some of the most gruesome human bodies imaginable—mangled, mutilated, crushed, or burned to a crisp.

Just as often, I would find myself visiting a nursing home instead of the hospital ER. The demographics of the area dictated that these homes were expensive and, therefore, well maintained—clean, flooded with sunshine, pleasant-smelling. The "guests" were always well cared for—bathed, perfumed, coiffed, sitting in clean rooms or clean sheets. Yet, I hated going to those nursing homes. But I did not mind going to the ER.

Sick? Psycho? Warped? Just the opposite. When I went into the ER, deep in my soul I knew there was a very slim chance that I would ever end up this way. I wasn't going to drive so recklessly that I would wrap myself around a telephone pole. I wasn't running with a crowd that dealt in murders. I was young and fast enough that I could run away from fiery flames. No. There was not a chance that I would end up here on the ER table, fighting for my life. I was too young, too strong, and essentially indestructible.

But when I entered the nursing home, deep in my soul I knew I had a real chance of ending up like this! I *realized* it. And that scared me. The chances I saw, way off in my future, but *my* future nonetheless, were that some day I would grow too old to take care of myself, that all my family would be unable to take care of me, that

I would end up stuck away in some "home." A terrible thought. A sad, lonely, frightening, humiliating vision.

Today, I kid my wife about the days when I might be feeble and mostly unable. Take me to the beach, I pray. Just stick me there with my iPod and let me watch the endless surf. Give me gentle love songs and rich, full orchestral extravaganzas. The music, the breeze, the warmth of the sun, the rhythmic dance of the ocean—this is all I will need. Yes, ideally that would be wonderful. But in the real world, that probably will not happen for a host of reasons.

Being in the fact-based world, I do fear the real possibility that this body will deteriorate to the point that I become like my mother-in-law is today. The disease need not be Alzheimer's, but any one of its many resemblances.

I fear being robbed of my self. Self will change, but today I don't want to look forward to a self that resembles Mom. And her sickness reminds me of this every day. It reminds me of my own eventual lack of control. It reminds me of the odds of becoming senile. It reminds me of realistic eventualities.... that I will be stuck in bed until someone comes and dresses me; that I will lose my freedom to come and go as I wish; that I will have days of excruciating frustration because I can not force my mind to think rationally; that I will have days of hollow emptiness because a single day will be recognized as 1,440 minutes lived for no purpose whatsoever; that there will be no hope for tomorrow because the very concept of "tomorrow" will have no meaning.

Perhaps there is a single blessing in Alzheimer's: eventually it shuts down your mind so you cannot understand how terrible it is and how terrible things are! Sometimes I really look at Mom, watch her, stare at her, and try to understand what's going on in her mind. I don't have a clue. But often I guess, "Nothing's going on." And I see that as a blessing for her.

But when I project it all to my own future, it scares me. I don't want that. I fear that.

A Prayer for Faith

I'm afraid, Lord.

I don't live in fear because I don't dwell on my frailty and mortality. But when I do think of these, I am afraid. I don't know whether my fear of getting sick, old, or feeble is more a lack of faith or too much pride. I know my pride makes me shrink at the image of being unable and needy. But worse yet is my lack of faith in your promise to watch over me, even more than you do the birds of the air.

Renew in me the gift of faith, Lord. I need to be reminded that you constantly are looking out for me, caring for me. I need to remind myself that I am in the palm of your hand. Today, when I look out the window, whether I see a sparrow or a dark cloud with nourishing rain, I will remember that you will provide for me. When I look at Mom, I will be reminded that you are the ultimate caregiver, and in your own wonderful and magnificent way you will provide for her and for me. When I feed

Mom, I will know that you nourish me with your love and your strength. I will know that no task is too large, no burden too heavy, with you at my side.

Renew my faith, Lord. Renew my trust in you.

Amen.

The Rewards

● ●

I have always considered myself a man of hope. I believe strongly in hope. Sometimes I think it is the greatest of virtues. Hope sees the positive in any and every situation. Hope begets comfort, strength, perseverance, and even joy. Hope helps us find rewards in even the darkest of places.

MY REWARDS

There are rich rewards to taking care of an Alzheimer's parent, spouse, or in-law. I made a list of the rewards I have noticed over the last few years, as well as asking Penny for a list. Let me start with what I see as blessings that have come out of this experience.

- ## Blessing #1
  ### My wife, the caregiver

The greatest gift I receive is to see daily the face of God in my wife. Penny is the primary caregiver in every sense. First, she made a commitment to take care of her mother and never pack her off to a home. This is pure love. She herself *takes care* of her mother. More than just providing for her, she cares for her, ministers to her, lays hands on her in a dozen wonderful blessings every day: feeds her, takes her to the bathroom, bathes her, puts make up on her, brushes her hair, cheers her up, takes her out, talks to her, reads to her, walks with her, encourages her. Conscious, constant love, love without hesitation, love never measured but always fully poured out, one-way love that seeks no reciprocity—simple, genuine, caring love. I am blessed to witness this every single day. It is not only a sign of my wife's magnificence. To me, it is a sign of God, a reminder of how he loves.

- Blessing #2
  My children, growing in character

I've always loved my children and my grandchildren. In my own prejudiced way, I have always judged them to be terrific (not perfect, but terrific!). But now I observe them growing in wisdom and love as they deal with this experience of Alzheimer's in our home. Mom's sickness has given them a unique opportunity to blossom; it has given me an opportunity to observe and enjoy that maturing love. I feel deep admiration for Emily when she comes over to our house to "baby-sit" her grandmother. She hugs her, sits with her, shows her pretty pictures in magazines, and talks to her with kindness and love in her voice. It is rewarding to see Jill come over most Monday mornings to help Penny take care of her mother. She gets her grandmother dressed and fed, or she might do household chores that otherwise Penny would have to do. Whatever she does, it is real help, comes with generosity, and is satisfying to watch. Jim comes over, always with his laptop, and takes a different approach. With real love he, more than anyone, challenges his grandmother, asking her questions, helping explain the answers to her, trying to push her to use the mental capacities that still exist. This is wonderful for me to witness my children, each in his or her own way showing the love they have for their grandmother. Her sickness, while negative in itself, attracts them back to our home where we can witness their love and take joy in their unselfish giving. This is an unintended reward; this is a blessing. *They* are a blessing.

Even with the grandchildren, I receive extra blessings as they give, in their own way, to their great grandmother. It is a real pleasure to watch Caroline, the very picture of caring. When she comes to help with Mom, she exhibits a calm, dedicated willingness to care for her in any and every way—feed her, take her to the bathroom, assist her in struggling through simple jigsaw puzzles—whatever is needed or helpful. I take pleasure in watching Christian grow in his understanding of sickness, old age, and caregiving. He has moved from indifference to leaving his Xbox and escorting Mom to the table for dinner. This is typical childlike love and comforting to watch. Even little Catherine—when she comes over to our house, she wants to run up and soothe Mom with lotion for her hands, arms, and feet. Their father, my son-in-law, always treats Mom to a dose of his inimitable dry humor. I find happiness in seeing each of my family prove that they understand the value of people over things, the value of giving over receiving, the value of love over self absorption.

- ### Blessing #3
  ### The opportunity to prepare for my future

Partly in jest, partly in wishful thinking, I have said for years that as long as I can continue kidding myself into believing that I am young, healthy, and fit, there will continue to be great joy in my life. A strong believer in mind-over-matter, I know this is true to a certain degree. But now, confronting Mom's sickness every day, I think I'm becoming a little more realistic about my own future.

Years ago, I told everyone that I am never going to die. That was a mixture of religious belief (I believe in the afterlife), youthful bravado, avoidance, and arrogance. Now I still believe in afterlife, but also I am willing to admit that this body of mine will die. Dealing with Alzheimer's in my house gives me the opportunity and the invitation to contemplate my own mortality and prepare for my own future. Since I'm still working, it is easy to stay busy and neglect to face life's more serious questions. But seeing "slow death" every day forces me to acknowledge human mortality, which, in turn, pushes me to consider the true value of my own life. I recognize for myself what I read recently: "What will matter is not my success, but my significance; not my competence, but my character." Mom's future is pretty well out of her hands. But I still have the time and talent for shaping my future, concentrating on significance, building my character, and preparing for my final years.

Without Alzheimer's in my life, I might just continue driving hard with little or no thought to where I am going and the significance of it all. But Mom's being with us blesses me with questions that need answers:

- Am I trying to be significant or merely successful?

- Am I still building my character or just my competence?

- Am I a man of integrity, true to my self and my values?

- If my mind just starts to evaporate, somehow lost in the fog of Alzheimer's, will someone still be left a better person because of my life and influence?

- When my body finally just goes away, will those I love look back on my life with pride and satisfaction?

Caring for an Alzheimer's patient forces one to consider the value of life and provides the opportunity to improve that life. As you confront another's death, you confront your own life. This truly is a gift, a blessing.

A Prayer in Appreciation

I give thanks to you, O God, for the magnificence of your creation.
I give thanks to you, for your great love is without end.

I thank you for Mom, who has brought a common focus and centeredness to this family.
I thank you for Penny, who shows me daily the meaning of gentle, loving service.
I thank you for my children, as I witness their growth in wisdom and grace.
I thank you for my grandchildren, as I watch them grow not just in body, but in spirit.

I thank you for my life—its past wonders, present joys and future promises.
I thank you for the hundred blessings I receive each day.
You are good to me, Lord. You are good to me.

Amen.

Penny's List

● ●

Penny's list is more beautiful than mine. When I asked her what rewards come from having her mother live with us, she said, "It gives me a chance to say good-bye to her every day—to tell her the things I always wanted to tell her but never did."

Such a tender and beautiful insight. Too often, when a parent dies, it happens suddenly. My dad just died, unexpectedly to me, my mother, and even his doctor. I did not have the gift of being able to say good-bye every day. This most important and highly influential person to me was abruptly ripped from my life. I didn't have the chance to say, "I love you…Thank you…Daddy, I've always wanted to tell that I really admired you when I came to watch you argue a case at the Hall of Justice." All my life I have missed something about my dad since he died. I missed more than him the person, my father. There was something else—*about* him, *special* to him, pertaining to him and me. I never understood what it was until Penny mentioned this unique blessing of an on-going good-bye. What I had missed all those years was the *processing* of my father's death, the *gradual* saying goodbye. I'm not talking about the mourning and grieving at and after death. I'm talking about the lead-up to death, the positive presence where two loving people can comfortably prepare for and peacefully experience parting—indeed a blessing. And specifically a blessing for a caregiver.

Penny pointed to a second reward she sees in her mother being with us. "It is a good way to honor my father and mother. I honor her every day now by caring for her. But I also honor Pop, who is the one who adored her and always took care of her."

Anyone who knows Penny will understand her complete love and admiration for her Pop. This was a man filled with passion, fun, adventure, and love. To him family, his wife and children, always came first. And he did "adore and take care of" his wife. He brought her breakfast in bed every day. He showed his love in a hundred ways every day. He was dedicated to his children—not just good *to* them, but good *for* them. He spent an unusual amount of time with his family because he wanted to, and because he put himself in a position to. By his own example he taught his children love, dedication, and service. Penny learned from him, in many ways emulates him. And there is no doubt that she honors him, his values, and his example by taking care of her mother, his wife. It is the finest tribute she can give him, imitating this most thoughtful man, her father.

Another gift that my wife senses in her caretaking is the ability to give back. "Taking care of her every day is my way to respond to the wonderful gifts she gave me—life, birth, education, love."

This is a direct "thank you." So often we take our parents for granted, especially in our own older age. We don't need them for room, board, or guidance. Certainly we don't spontaneously feel gratitude for our birth or education. But parents are, in fact, the source. They have been the givers of the most basic and wonderful gifts we have ever received. They never asked for payment in return, but daily care is as close a pay-back as we can give for the generous gifts they willingly bestowed on us.

"These are the three greatest gifts or rewards I see from all this," Penny told me. "There are others: giving the kids a chance to learn how to respect the elderly, fully appreciating the love of those friends who take the time to understand and support us, learning patience. And I realize that I'm doing the best I can; and when Mom dies, I'll have no regrets. These are the rewards I reap every day."

A Prayer for My Family

Bless my family, Lord—my wife, my children, my grandchildren. The family has always been a sign of your divine being and your love. I thank you for this most special blessing in my life. My wife, my children, my grandchildren all bring me joy. Sure, there are times when I could strangle them, but abundant joy is the dominant feeling, the recognized gift, and the normal blessing of being with them.

I thank God for the happiness and laughter of my grandchildren. I appreciate their growing in intelligence and knowledge as they go through school. But it is their smiles and young laughter that most make me happy.

I thank you for my children—mature, smart, and coping with the challenges of the world. It is a blessing for me to have them all an integral part of my life; a blessing that I can be with them so often. They give me new insights into your universe, Lord, opening to me new interpretations of life that I would never have seen on my own.

Finally, you know that I thank you for my wife. She is, to me, a sign of your love—unselfish, constant, and freely given. Outside of your grace, she is the greatest gift you have given me. I thank you for her each and every day of my life.

Amen.

What If I Get Alzheimer's?

● ●

I mentioned earlier in this book that I fear I could get Alzheimer's. I choose to believe that it is not likely, but it is possible just as it is possible to get dementia and suffer from that. Thinking about it, I have developed some preferences for my life at that stage. I write this chapter now to my children in hopes that they read it again if and when I get Alzheimer's.

• My Wishes

I want my wife and children each to have their own life.

I know my wife and children will always love me even if I am sick, no matter how sick I am. The love that we taught our kids, the example of love, and caregiving that we (mostly Penny) have shown them—these could put a burden on the children to follow our example and take us into their own home. But I do not want my children to take me into their homes to care for me. I want them, if at all possible, to get care for me in other ways. With my long-term care insurance, I can be in a nursing home or they can get professional help to take care of me in my own house.

I want them to have a rich life where they can focus on their own relationships, agenda, and priorities. I don't want my illness to be a constant drain on them. I don't want them setting their daily agenda around me and my needs. I don't want them losing sleep every night because they are half-awake listening for my needing them. Simply, I want the priority of their time, their health, and their attention to be directed to their own lives—not mine.

Sure, I will want to see them, hear them, and have them hold my hand and assure me. I will want their attention and comfort. But it is their turn now to live their own lives. As much as I love them, cherish them, and appreciate them, *because* I love them, I do not want to demand an inordinate amount of their attention.

I want my children to remember that I love them.

I'm sure I will provide more frustration to my children than Mom does to me. I'm opinionated, outspoken, and stubborn. I suspect I will be a handful if I get to the point that Mom is.

So kids, here is what I want you to realize:

- If I am grumpy and uncommunicative, it is only because my mind is not working correctly.

- If I do not say, "Thank you," it is only because I no longer understand gratitude.

- If I am rude or neglectful, it is only because I no longer realize what common courtesy is.

- If I forget what you just told me, it is because my memory has shut down.

- If I do what you just told me not to do, it is because I never comprehended your instruction.

- If I look at you with a blank stare, it is because I am living with a blank mind.

- If I ignore you, it is because I don't have the mental strength to comprehend your presence.

- But know that I love you and will love you always to the best of my capacity and my ability. Know that, when the time is right, I will personally ask God, who created each of us, to repay you one hundred fold for all you have given me.

For myself, I think I will want music, laughter and …

Admittedly, there is some fantasy in these next several paragraphs. I've witnessed enough Alzheimer's to understand that anyone with this disease does not get to determine the day's schedule. Independence is gone; one becomes subjugated to another's will and schedule; decisions about where you will be and how you will spend your days are made by others. If I ever have Alzheimer's or dementia, I probably won't know what I will want or appreciate. But if I am allowed a dream or two about my own future with Alzheimer's, this is it:

I think I will want to be left alone a lot. I don't think I will want people, even people I love, constantly telling me what to do, where to go, or how to act. Today, I even think I might want everyone to just let me die! I might change this wish if I do, in fact, get to the point of having Alzheimer's. But right now, this one makes sense—let me die.

Actually, when I really think about it, there might be a way I would like to continue living–even with this terrible disease. If you can arrange it, prop me daily in a comfortable lounge chair at the beach. Not good for skin cancer, but by that point, why worry about skin cancer? I want to hear the constant, mesmerizing rhythm of the ocean, see the silver and gold shimmer of sunlight atop the vast blue waterbed of the sea, feel the warm, weathering wind against my cheeks, and smell the rich aroma wafting off the life-filled waters.

I want to hear also the music of my iPod—sometimes soft, gentle, and romantic; sometimes loud, robust, and fully orchestral.

I will want to hear laughter. So when you drag me back into my room, put on a DVD of the Three Stooges or Abbott and Costello or the entire Pink Panther series. Of course, to go with my video and laughter, a bowl of rich, smooth chocolate ice cream. Or peppermint will be fine. And before dinner, a sip of Maker's Mark.

Thank You for Worldly Pleasures

Thank you for the gifts that make me glad, Lord. The wonderful, worldly, and physical pleasures that thrill my senses.

Thank you for the beach. To me it has always been a vision of power and glory. Thank you for the endless vista of water, extending to that line where sky meets sea.

Thank you for the feel of mildly coarse sand scraping the skin of my feet. Thank you for the calming, rhythmic, and muffled roar of salt-heavy water rolling onto the sand. Thank you for the primal taste of salt that dusts my lips. Thank you for the lusty smell at water's edge where Triton deposits traces of his treasures.

Thank you for Beethoven and the Beatles, rap and rhapsodies, concerts and cantatas. Thank you for that good 'ol rock n' roll where the music soothes my soul. Thank you for Gregorian chant, which places me vividly in your presence. Thank you for the sweet sounds of the flute and the bold slurs of the trombone.

Thank you for laughter. The delighted giggle of a little child, the hearty response to a good joke, and the sustained chuckles at a comedian's routine. Thank you for my funny bone and a sense of humor. Thank you for Marcel and Johnny and Seinfeld.

And thank you for good food—be it a rich, double-chocolate Fenton's milkshake, a Colonial French-cruller donut, a lusty chimichanga, a grilled, fresh salmon steak, or a magnificent Oakville cab.

These are simple pleasures, Lord. Ultimately, they all come from you, the Creator. So, to you, with obvious simplicity but true sincerity, I say: Thank you.

Amen.

Is There Hope?

There *always* is hope.

• Simply, Yes. There Is Hope

When Penny's mom came to live with us, we were clueless about what this visit would become. We knew she was getting old, getting a little feebler, and slowing down mentally; but we had no real appreciation of what her sickness would do to her life and ours. The reality of it all shocked me into a heavy case of resentment at first. It was easy to see everything negative about this entire situation—Alzheimer's the sickness, Mom moving in, the change of priorities and schedules, the strain on my wife, and the apparent squeeze on our freedom or certainly our normal schedule. All those negative feelings—they were real, daily, imposing, eating at my soul.

I've always said that feelings are fair. So my resentments and anger were all fair as far as feelings go. But time helps us change our definitions of normal, fair, and okay. In time, the situation of Mom living with us somehow became normal, fair, and okay. Believe this, my friend. Just the very thought of this will help you at the beginning. It will give you hope.

Early on, things may seem bad. And they are, but it will get better. You will change, find new insights, and shift some focus off yourself so that the willingness to focus on your sick parent increases.

The negatives morph into the ordinary.

The "Why are we doing this!" in time becomes "I'm glad we're doing this because it is the noble thing to do."

You no longer miss your old routines of going out to dinner or a movie.

You'll enjoy a deeper love with the few friends who really try to understand what you're dealing with.

You'll understand that your spouse still loves you every bit as much as ever, perhaps even more so.

Most importantly, you'll recognize that you have lost nothing of your self, but have actually grown in character.

Previously, I summed up my early frustrations with this statement: "I want my house back. I want my wife back. I want my life back." Well, I have them back. I have them back because I had hope. I have them back because of the strong trust and love between my wife and myself. I have them back because of our daily commitment to care for Mom. I have them back because, with my wife's understanding and encouragement, I have made duty and love overcome my frustrations and anger.

There is hope because life is not static.

There is hope because you can decide your own attitudes.

There is hope because you can choose to become a greater lover and servant.

There is hope because each day you can choose how you will react to the realities of this one day.

There is hope because there are others who will help you, guide you, and support you as long as you are willing to ask.

There is hope because God's grace is generous and he willingly gives you as much of his grace as you want.

If you are a Christian, you are familiar with the Gospel of the Talents. God gets angry at those who have talents but refuse to use them and expect him to do all the work for us. God gives us his grace, but he expects us to work to make things happen. The real basis of my hope is God's power and gifts. But I support that hope and respond to it by working to improve my self, my life, my environment, my choices, and my responses.

I recommend that you read again the chapter on coping skills. Utilize them or find your own coping skills. Use your talents to make life more positive and fulfilling. You owe that to yourself, even while you care daily for another.

A Prayer of Hope

You are the source of my hope, Lord. For anyone who takes the time to think of your life, there is hope. Even short of anything as phenomenal as the Resurrection, there is incredible hope for anyone who looks at your life.

There was a man possessed with evil spirits. You said, "Be quiet and come out of him." And he was relieved of those evil spirits. There is hope for me, Lord!

Simon's mother-in-law was sick with a fever. They asked you to cure her. You did. Then they brought hundreds of sick to you. You placed your hands on every one of them and healed them. There is hope for me, Lord!

They let a paralyzed man down from the roof opening to set him at your feet. You healed him. There is hope for me, Lord.

You healed the man with the withered hand, the blind man, the woman hemorrhaging, the ruler's son, and the ten lepers. There is hope for me, Lord!

My problems are not physical. They are more emotional and spiritual—a lack of trust, a lack of patience, a lack of generosity, a lack of kindness. These add up to a lack of love. So my prayer must be: Fill me with your love, Lord. Let me grow in love. I have hope that daily I can grow into this role of caregiver. I can become better and better day by day; more kind, solicitous, patient, and giving. I know I can become better and better in this environment. And I believe that, with your grace, I will.

I live in hope, Lord. Prove me right.

Amen.

Epilogue

● ●

This book was written for you, the caretaker, or the spouse of a caretaker. I focused on the caring of an Alzheimer's patient. But the basic ideas in this book apply to anyone having difficulty in constantly caring for any sick person with any overwhelming sickness.

I've taken a few liberties with the accuracy of describing some events. Usually, I do this so as not to embarrass someone. At other times, I have combined several facts or incidents into a single story for the sake of brevity or simplicity. But the sense of what I write is always true to my feelings.

I write as one living with an Alzheimer's patient in my home. I am not the primary caregiver; my wife is. The patient is her mother, not mine. As the secondary caregiver, the in-law, I recognize that I have it relatively easy. I have enormous respect for those who are the primary caregivers. Their emotions must be more tempestuous than mine, many the same, many different, but a wide range of emotions nonetheless.

I share my own kaleidoscope of emotions to warn you about what you will face. I share my story so you can realize that you are not alone, that others understand exactly what you are going through. I include my prayers because they express my soul, and may find a soul-mate in you. I explain my coping tools in the hope that you will use them or something similar to cope with your situation

Make life as good as it can be for your self. While you watch a loved one die, you can in fact make your own life more significant and noble.

Do so.

THERE IS HELP

To keep in touch with other caregivers, to ask them questions, to share your frustrations, suggestions and successes, go online to: caregiverconnect.blogspot.com

To contact the Alzheimer's Association,
visit: www.alz.org

For information about having the author speak to your organization or group, please send an e-mail to: joe@skillinmarketing.com